Table of Contents

10 Ways to Boost Male Fertility and Increase Sperm Count

If you and your partner are experiencing fertility issues, know that you're not alone. Infertility is more common than you might think.

It affects about one in every six couples, and researchers estimate about one in every three cases is due to fertility problems in the male partner alone.

While infertility is not always treatable, there are some things you can do to boost your chances of conceiving. Fertility can sometimes be improved with a healthy diet, supplements, and other lifestyle strategies.

This book lists some of the main lifestyle factors, foods, nutrients, and supplements that have been associated with improved fertility in men.

What is male infertility?

Fertility refers to people's ability to reproduce without medical assistance.

Male infertility is when a man has a poor chance of making his female partner pregnant. It usually depends on the quality of his sperm cells.

Sometimes infertility is linked to sexual function, and other times it could be linked to semen quality. Here are some examples of each:

- **Libido.** Otherwise known as sex drive, libido describes a person's desire to have sex. Foods or supplements that claim to increase libido are called aphrodisiacs.

- **Erectile dysfunction.** Also known as impotence, erectile dysfunction is when a man is unable to develop or maintain an erection.

- **Sperm count.** An important aspect of semen quality is the number or concentration of sperm cells in a given amount of semen.

- **Sperm motility.** An essential function of healthy sperm cells is their ability to swim. Sperm motility is measured as the percentage of moving sperm cells in a sample of semen.

- **Testosterone levels.** Low levels of testosterone, the male sex hormone, may be responsible for infertility in some men.

Infertility can have multiple causes and may depend on genetics, general health, fitness, diseases, and dietary contaminants.

Additionally, a healthy lifestyle and diet are important. Some foods and nutrients are associated with greater fertility benefits than others.

Here are 10 science-backed ways to boost sperm count and increase fertility in men.

1. Take D-aspartic acid supplements

D-aspartic acid (D-AA) is a form of aspartic acid, a type of amino acid that's sold as a dietary supplement.

It should not be confused with L-aspartic acid, which makes up the structure of many proteins and is far more common than D-AA.

D-AA is mainly present in certain glands, such as the testicles, as well as in semen and sperm cells.

Researchers believe that D-AA is implicated in male fertility. In fact, D-AA levels are significantly lower in infertile men than fertile men.

This is supported by studies showing that D-AA supplements may increase levels of testosterone, the male sex hormone that plays an essential role in male fertility.

For example, a study in infertile men suggested that taking 2.7 grams of D-

AA for 3 months increased their testosterone levels by 30–60% and sperm count and motility by 60–100%.

The number of pregnancies also increased among their partners (4).

Another controlled study in healthy men showed that taking 3 grams of D-AA supplements daily for 2 weeks increased testosterone levels by 42%.

However, the evidence is not consistent. Studies in athletes or strength-trained men with normal to high testosterone levels found that D-

AA didn't increase its levels further and even reduced them at high doses.

The current evidence indicates that D-AA supplements may improve fertility in men with low testosterone levels, while they don't consistently provide additional benefits in men with normal to high levels.

More research is needed to investigate the potential long-term risks and benefits of D-AA supplements in humans.

2. Exercise regularly

Besides being good for your general health, exercising regularly can boost testosterone levels and improve fertility.

Studies show that men who exercise regularly have higher testosterone levels and better semen quality than inactive men.

However, you should avoid too much exercise, as it may have the opposite effect and potentially reduce testosterone levels. Getting the right amount of zinc can minimize this risk.

If you rarely exercise but want to improve your fertility, make becoming physically active one of your top priorities.

3. Get enough vitamin C

You're probably familiar with vitamin C's ability to boost the immune system.

Some evidence indicates that taking antioxidant supplements, such as vitamin C, may improve fertility.

Oxidative stress is when levels of reactive oxygen species (ROS) reach harmful levels in the body.

It happens when the body's own antioxidant defenses are overwhelmed because of disease, old age, an unhealthy lifestyle, or environmental pollutants.

ROS are constantly being produced in the body, but their levels are kept in check in healthy people. High levels of ROS may promote tissue injury and inflammation, increasing the risk of chronic disease.

There's also some evidence that oxidative stress and excessively high levels of ROS may lead to infertility in men.

Taking in enough antioxidants, such as vitamin C, may help counteract some of these harmful effects. There's also some evidence that vitamin C supplements may improve semen quality.

A study in infertile men showed that taking 1,000-mg vitamin C supplements twice a day for up to 2 months increased sperm motility by 92% and sperm count by more than

100%. It also reduced the proportion of deformed sperm cells by 55%.

Another observational study in Indian industrial workers suggested that taking 1,000 mg of vitamin C five times a week for 3 months may protect against DNA damage caused by ROS in sperm cells.

Vitamin C supplements also significantly improved sperm count and motility, while reducing the numbers of deformed sperm cells.

Taken together, these findings suggest that vitamin C may help improve fertility in infertile men with oxidative stress.

However, controlled studies are needed before any definite claims can be made.

4. Relax and minimize stress

It's hard to get in the mood when you're feeling stressed, but there might be more to it than not feeling up for sex. Stress may reduce your sexual satisfaction and impair your fertility.

Researchers believe the hormone cortisol may partly explain these adverse effects of stress.

Prolonged stress raises levels of cortisol, which has strong negative effects on testosterone. When cortisol goes up, testosterone levels tend to go down.

While severe, unexplained anxiety is typically treated with medication, milder forms of stress can be reduced with relaxation techniques.

Stress management can be as simple as taking a walk in nature, meditating, exercising, or spending time with friends.

5. Get enough vitamin D

Vitamin D can be important for male and female fertility. It's another nutrient that may boost testosterone levels.

One observational study showed that vitamin-D-deficient men were more likely to have low testosterone levels.

A controlled study in 65 men with low testosterone levels and vitamin D deficiency supported these findings. Taking 3,000 IU of vitamin D3 every day for 1 year increased their testosterone levels by around 25%.

High vitamin D levels are linked to greater sperm motility, but the evidence is inconsistent.

6. Try tribulus terrestris

Tribulus terrestris, also known as puncture vine, is a medicinal herb frequently used to enhance male fertility.

One study in men with low sperm counts showed that taking 6 grams of tribulus root twice daily for 2 months improved erectile function and libido.

While Tribulus terrestris does not raise testosterone levels, research indicates that it may enhance the libido-promoting effects of testosterone.

However, further studies are needed to confirm its aphrodisiac properties and evaluate the long-term risks and benefits of supplementing with it.

7. Take fenugreek supplements

Fenugreek (Trigonella foenum-graecum) is a popular culinary and medicinal herb.

One study in 30 men who strength-trained four times a week analyzed the effects of taking 500 mg of fenugreek extract daily.

The men experienced significantly increased testosterone levels, strength, and fat loss, compared with a placebo.

Another study in 60 healthy men showed that taking 600 mg of Testofen, a supplement made from fenugreek seed extract and minerals, daily for 6 weeks improved libido, sexual performance, and strength.

These findings were confirmed by another, larger study in 120 healthy men. Taking 600 mg of Testofen every day for 3 months improved self-reported erectile function and the frequency of sexual activity.

Also, the supplement significantly increased testosterone levels.

Keep in mind that all of these studies examined fenugreek extracts. It's unlikely that whole fenugreek, which is used in cooking and herbal tea, is as effective.

8. Get enough zinc

Zinc is an essential mineral found in high amounts in animal foods, such as meat, fish, eggs, and shellfish.

Getting enough zinc is one of the cornerstones of male fertility.

Observational studies show that low zinc status or deficiency is associated with low testosterone levels, poor sperm quality, and an increased risk of male infertility.

Also, taking zinc supplements increases testosterone levels and sperm count in those who are low in zinc.

Furthermore, zinc supplements may reduce the decreased testosterone levels that are associated with excessive amounts of high-intensity exercise.

Controlled trials need to confirm these observational findings.

9. Consider ashwagandha

Ashwagandha (Withania somnifera) is a medicinal herb that's been used in India since ancient times.

Studies suggest that ashwagandha may improve male fertility by boosting testosterone levels.

One study in men with low sperm cell counts showed that taking 675 mg of ashwagandha root extract per day for

3 months significantly improved fertility.

Specifically, it increased sperm counts by 167%, semen volume by 53%, and sperm motility by 57%, compared with levels at the start of the study. In comparison, minimal improvements were detected among those who got a placebo treatment.

Increased testosterone levels may be partly responsible for these benefits.

A study in 57 young men following a strength-training program showed that consuming 600 mg of ashwagandha root extract daily significantly increased testosterone levels, muscle mass, and strength, compared with a placebo.

These findings are supported by observational evidence indicating that ashwagandha supplements may improve sperm counts, sperm motility, antioxidant status, and testosterone levels.

10. Eat maca root

Taking maca root supplements may improve libido, as well as fertility and sexual performance.

Maca root is a popular plant food that originated in central Peru. Traditionally, it has been used for its ability to enhance libido and fertility.

Several studies in men showed that taking 1.5–3 grams of dried maca root for periods of up to 3 months improved self-reported sexual desire or libido.

Studies also suggest that maca root may improve sexual performance. In men with mild erectile dysfunction, taking 2.4 grams of dried maca root for 12 weeks slightly improved self-reported erectile function and sexual well-being.

Taking 1.75 grams of maca root powder every day for 3 months also increased sperm count and motility in healthy men.

These findings have been partly confirmed by reviews, but the researchers noted that the evidence is weak and more research is needed before definite claims can be made.

Additionally, maca root doesn't seem to affect hormone levels. Taking 1.5–3 grams of maca root per day for 3 months had no effects on testosterone or other reproductive hormones in healthy, fertile men.

Other tips

Many things can help boost fertility, but what works for you depends on the cause of your fertility issues.

Also, keep in mind that fertility and libido usually go hand in hand with your general health.

For this reason, anything that improves your overall health is likely to boost your fertility.

Here are 8 additional tips to boost fertility and sperm count/quality:

- **Lead a healthy lifestyle.** Unhealthy lifestyle practices impair your overall health, including fertility.

- **Lose excess weight.** Carrying extra weight is associated with infertility. If your doctor suspects that weight may be linked to your infertility, discuss weight loss as one of your health goals.

- **Limit your alcohol intake.** Avoid heavy alcohol consumption, as it may reduce testosterone levels and impair semen quality.

- **Get enough folate.** A few studies indicate that a low intake of folate may impair semen quality.

- **Get adequate sleep.** Getting adequate sleep is vital to maintaining your health. Restricted or excessive sleep has also been linked to poor semen quality.

- Snack on walnuts. Eating a lot of antioxidant-rich foods, such as walnuts, seems to benefit fertility.

- **Consider supplements.** Antioxidant supplements also seem to work. Some evidence suggests that coenzyme Q10 improves semen quality.

- **Avoid eating too much soy.** Soy is rich in isoflavones, which are associated with lower semen quality.

The bottom line

Infertility is fairly common and affects many men worldwide.

If you're having fertility issues, one thing you can do is focus on improving your general health. Many of the tips mentioned above are key components of a healthy lifestyle.

There's no guaranteed fix, but if nutrient deficiencies or low testosterone levels are contributing factors, chances are that these lifestyle tips may help.

Does Alcohol Kill Sperm? And Other Fertility Facts

When it comes to alcohol and fertility, the focus is quite often on the woman.

We know about the harmful effects of drinking while pregnant, but what about drinking before pregnancy? And how does drinking affect male fertility? Is it a big deal? Should you even worry about it?

Yes, you should.

Alcohol, even in moderate amounts, can affect your sexual health. It can lead to loss of libido and infertility in both men and women.

Read on to learn how alcohol affects sperm and male and female fertility.

How much alcohol does it take to affect sperm and male fertility?

Social alcohol use is common around the world, but heavy drinking has lots of bad health effects. In the United States, a 2015 survey found nearly 27 percent of those 18 or older reported binge drinking in the past month.

According to the Centers for Disease Control and Prevention (CDC), in approximately 35 percent of cases of infertility, male and female factors were identified.

Studies show heavy, consistent drinking or binge drinking — five or more drinks in men in a two-hour timeframe — have negative effects on sperm.

More than 14 mixed drinks in a week can lower testosterone levels and affect sperm count.

How alcohol affects sperm and male fertility

The bad news

Alcohol can affect fertility by altering sperm count, size, shape, and motility.

In men, heavy drinking affects fertility by:

- lowering testosterone levels, follicle stimulating hormone, and luteinizing hormone, and raising estrogen levels, which reduce sperm production

- shrinking the testes, which can cause impotence or infertility

• changing gonadotropin release which impacts sperm production

• causing early ejaculation or decreased ejaculation

• changing the shape, size, and movement of healthy sperm

Combining drugs like marijuana or opioids with alcohol also lowers fertility. In addition, liver disease caused by excessive drinking can change sperm quality.

Moreover, recent animal and human studies show exposure to alcohol during early development and later in life leads to changes in the DNA. This, in turn, may lead to alcohol use disorder and other inherited health problems. More research, however, is needed to confirm this connection.

The good news

The effects of alcohol on sperm count are reversible.

The good news is that the effects are reversible. One study showed it took three months for the return of healthy sperm production once alcohol consumption stops.

How alcohol affects female fertility

Alcohol can lower the chances of becoming pregnant.

According to a recent study, regular heavy drinking can reduce female fertility by:

- interrupting menstrual cycle and ovulation causing changes to ovarian function, known as amenorrhea and anovulation, respectively

- changing hormone levels of testosterone, estradiol and luteinizing hormone

- causing hyperprolactinemia or high prolactin in the blood

Studies also confirm alcohol exposure during pregnancy is harmful. Fetal alcohol spectrum disorders are one example of a side effect.

How to boost male fertility

A healthy lifestyle is a crucial part of boosting fertility. Excessive drinking, stress, anxiety, being overweight, and smoking can all hurt your health and fertility.

A new study found those who consumed a healthy Mediterranean diet had higher sperm quality. This was especially true for those eating more fruits, vegetables, seafood, and healthy grains.

Tips for increasing male fertility

- exercising regularly to boost testosterone levels

- practicing stress management to keep cortisol levels down

- follow good sleep habits

- discuss your nutritional needs with your doctor to find out if you're low on any vitamins

When to see a doctor

Lifestyle, medications, and hormonal or genetic conditions can all play a role in infertility. Typically, a male hormone analysis and semen analysis can help identify underlying issues.

You can also try home test kits. However, these kits will only tell you sperm count. They don't tell you about other possible reasons for infertility such as quality or movement of sperm.

It's best to speak to your doctor if you have concerns and are considering testing your sperm.

Whether you've been trying for a while or you're just starting to plan for a family, there's no time like the present to make some healthy lifestyle changes.

You can make a healthy start by:

- managing your weight

- following a healthy diet

- getting into a regular exercise routine

- practicing self-care

- quitting smoking and excessive drinking

- managing any chronic conditions, such as diabetes, high blood pressure, asthma, or other conditions

Schedule an appointment with your doctor to talk about any specific fertility concerns. Always talk to your pharmacist and doctor before you consider any over-the-counter vitamins or supplements.

5 Common Signs of Infertility in Men and Women

I was 26 years old when I was first diagnosed with infertility. In my case, the inability to conceive was the result of a condition called stage 4 endometriosis.

Like many people facing infertility, I was heartbroken by the news. I'd always believed I'd have a large family. The choices I found myself having to make in the years that followed, and the mounting agony of repeat in vitro fertilization (IVF) cycles, left me devastated.

It's common for couples to experience issues with infertility. Many of these couples have no symptoms. They don't have any reason to suspect they may have infertility until they start trying to conceive.

For this reason, it's recommended that couples who've been trying to get pregnant for over a year without success seek the advice of a doctor. For women over age 35, that timeline is reduced to six months. Infertility issues increase with age.

Signs and Symptoms of Infertility

Signs and symptoms of infertility are often related to other underlying conditions. For example, 10 to 15 percent of untreated chlamydia cases will lead to pelvic inflammatory disease (PID). PID leads to a blockage of the fallopian tubes, which prevents fertilization.

There are numerous conditions that can contribute to infertility in men and women. The signs and symptoms of each can vary greatly. If you're concerned, it's important to consult with your doctor.

Common Signs of Infertility in Women

1. Irregular periods

The average woman's cycle is 28 days long. But anything within a few days of that can be considered normal, as long as those cycles are consistent. For example, a woman who has a 33-day cycle one month, a 31-day cycle the next, and a 35-day cycle after that, is probably having "normal" periods.

But a woman whose cycles vary so greatly that she can't even begin to estimate when her period might arrive is experiencing irregular periods. This can be related to hormone issues, or to polycystic ovarian syndrome (PCOS). Both of these can contribute to infertility.

2. Painful or heavy periods

Most women experience cramps with their periods. But painful periods that interfere with your daily life may be a symptom of endometriosis.

3. No periods

It's not uncommon for women to have an off month here and there. Factors like stress or heavy workouts can cause your period to temporarily disappear. But if you haven't had a period in months, it's time to get your fertility checked.

4. Symptoms of hormone fluctuations

Signs of hormone fluctuations in women could indicate potential issues with fertility. Talk to your doctor if you experience the following:

- skin issues

- reduced sex drive

- facial hair growth

- thinning hair

- weight gain

5. Pain during sex

Some women have experienced painful sex their entire lives, so they've convinced themselves it's normal. But it's not. It could be related to hormone issues, to endometriosis, or to other underlying conditions that could also be contributing to infertility.

Common Signs of Infertility in Men

1. Changes in sexual desire

A man's fertility is also linked with his hormone health. Changes in virility, often governed by hormones, could indicate issues with fertility.

2. Testicle pain or swelling

There are several different conditions that could lead to pain or swelling in the testicles, many of which could contribute to infertility.

3. Problems maintaining erection

A man's ability to maintain an erection
is often linked to his hormone levels.
Reduced hormones may result, which
could potentially translate into trouble
conceiving.

4. Issues with ejaculation

Similarly, an inability to ejaculate is a
sign that it might be time to visit a
doctor.

5. Small, firm testicles

The testes house a man's sperm, so
testicle health is paramount to male
fertility. Small or firm testicles could

indicate potential issues that should be explored by a medical practitioner.

The Takeaway

Around 15 to 20 percent of couples trying to conceive will have trouble with infertility. Female factor infertility is typically to blame 40 percent of the time, while male factor infertility is the cause of issues 30 to 40 percent of the time. A combination of these factors leads to infertility 20 to 30 percent of the time.

If you've been diagnosed with infertility, or fear you may have trouble conceiving in the future, you're not alone. The medical industry is forever making advances in this field. Make an appointment with your doctor and go over your concerns. Even if you are diagnosed with infertility, you may still be able to conceive.

What Is Sperm Motility and How Does It Affect Fertility?

Sperm health is an important factor in a couple's ability to conceive. There are six main criteria for healthy sperm:

- volume

- motility

- shape

- ability to pass through the cervical mucus and make it to the egg

- acrosome reaction

- zona pellucida binding

- nuclear decondensation

Sperm also need to have the right number of chromosomes for a successful pregnancy. A breakdown in any of these criteria can result in male-factor infertility.

An estimated 15–20 percent of couples worldwide are affected by infertility. Of those, approximately 30–40 percent are infertile due to male factors, including sperm motility. Another 20 percent are infertile due to a combination of male and female factors.

Sperm motility and pregnancy

Healthy sperm motility is defined as sperm with forward progressions of at least 25 micrometers per second. If a man has poor sperm mobility, it's called asthenospermia or asthenozoospermia. There are different types of sperm motility issues, including:

• slow or sluggish progressive motility

• non-progressive motility, which is defined as anything less than 5 micrometers per second

- no mobility

Sperm speed and gender: Fact or fiction?

It's long been thought that sperm with Y chromosomes, or "boy" sperm, swim faster than sperm with X chromosomes, known as "girl" sperm. Studies have proven that this is a myth, however, and there is no noticeable difference in motility or speed between X and Y sperm.

Causes

The exact cause for low sperm motility can vary. Some men may have a genetic cause, while others may have an undiagnosed medical condition. Lifestyle and environmental factors also play a big role in sperm motility. Smoking, for example, has been linked to decreased sperm motility, especially if the man smokes more than 10 cigarettes per day. Men who work in the military or have jobs that include painting, driving, or repeated trauma to the pelvic area may be at risk for work-induced infertility.

A condition called varicocele occurs when veins inside the scrotum become enlarged. This has also been linked to decreased sperm motility.

Low sperm motility may also be due to a disorder in the male accessory sex gland secretion, which leads to the glands emptying more slowly.

Diagnosis

Sperm motility can be tested through a routine semen analysis. For the test, you'll need to provide at least two semen samples. These are usually obtained by masturbation at a doctor's office or testing facility. It's also possible to obtain a sperm sample by having sex with a condom or withdrawing to obtain the sample. The sample must be kept at room temperature and delivered to the facility within 30 to 60 minutes. If less than 40 percent of your sperm are motile, your considered to have low sperm motility.

In addition to sperm motility, your doctor can also use a semen analysis to test:

• the health of the male genital tract

• accessory organs

• ejaculation

Treatment

Some lifestyle changes may help increase sperm motility for some men:

- exercise regularly

- maintain a healthy weight

- limit cell phone exposure

- reduce alcohol

- quit smoking

Some supplements may also help improve sperm motility. For example, one study found a 52 percent increase in sperm motility in men who took a daily supplement of 200 micrograms of selenium along with 400 units of vitamin E for at least 100 days in a row. Speak to your doctor before taking supplements, and be careful about where you buy them. Supplements are not regulated, so you should only buy them from reputable vendors.

If the cause of the sperm mobility issue is a medical problem, such as low hormone levels or varicocele, medication such as follicle-stimulating hormone or human chorionic gonadotropin may help. In some cases, your doctor may recommend surgery.

Outlook

Many factors can affect male fertility. If the sperm is otherwise healthy, pregnancy with low sperm motility can occur. Using a reproductive technology such as in vitro fertilization or intrauterine insemination (IUI) can help increase the chance of pregnancy. This is because they bypass the need for the sperm to swim on their own.

Talk to your doctor if you've been trying unsuccessfully to conceive for

12 or more months. Your doctor can test you and your partner to determine if there are any health conditions affecting fertility. Your doctor will then determine next steps.

7 Tips for Healthy Sperm

Overview

If you and your partner are trying to conceive a baby, you may be looking for information about how to increase sperm count to improve your chances of getting pregnant. A healthy sperm count is necessary for fertility.

For pregnancy to occur, only one sperm and one egg are needed, so why does sperm count matter? In short, it increases the odds for a successful pregnancy. When a man ejaculates into a woman, the chances that one sperm will reach and implant itself into an egg increases if more sperm are in the semen.

Normal semen contains 40 million to 300 million sperm per milliliter. A low sperm count is considered to be anything between 10 and 20 million sperm per milliliter. Twenty million sperm per milliliter may be adequate for pregnancy if the sperm are healthy.

Read on to learn more about sperm count plus seven things you can do to improve sperm health.

1. Lose weight

Losing weight if you're overweight is one of the single-most effective things you can do to increase sperm count. Studies have shown that weight loss can significantly increase semen volume, concentration, and mobility, as well as the overall health of sperm. The changes in sperm count have been found to be most significant in men who have a higher body mass index, so if you have a large amount of weight to lose, even losing a small amount of weight may help.

To accomplish your weight loss goals, talk to a doctor who can help you get started. You may want to schedule an appointment with a nutritionist to change any eating habits that could be improved. Working with a trainer or other exercise program can also help.

2. Exercise

Even if you don't need to lose weight, staying active and leading a healthy lifestyle can help boost your sperm count. One study found that weightlifting and outdoors exercise can help sperm health more than other types of exercise. Consider incorporating these kinds of activities into your routine. Exercise can also help you maintain or lose weight, which may have additional benefits for your sperm health.

3. Take your vitamins

Some types of vitamins, including vitamins D, C, E, and CoQ10, are important for sperm health.

One study showed that taking 1,000 mg of vitamin C every day can help men's sperm concentration and mobility. The overall sperm count won't improve, but the sperm can become more concentrated and able to move more efficiently. That can boost your chances of conceiving successfully.

Another study noted less successful rates of pregnancy among couples where the man had low levels of vitamin D. More research is needed to understand the relationship between this vitamin and fertility, but there does seem to be a correlation.

Talk to your doctor about testing your vitamin levels. They can do this using a simple blood test.

4. Avoid substance abuse

Low sperm counts and unhealthy sperm have been linked to people with a history of:

- heavy drinking, which is defined as drinking two or more alcoholic drinks per day

- tobacco use of any kind

- illegal drug use, including cocaine and anabolic steroids

If you use any of these substances and are having trouble quitting, talk to your doctor. They can recommend programs to help manage and treat addiction.

5. Check your environment

Consider changing your clothes and showering as soon as possible if you've been exposed to:

- metals

- solvents

- pesticides

- paint strippers

- degreasers

- non-water based glues or paints

- other endocrine disruptors

Those toxins may affect sperm count. If you're exposed to any of these things because of a hobby, consider putting your hobby on hold until after you've successfully conceived.

Jobs that expose you to excess heat or radiation, or even extreme sedentary work can also affect sperm count.

6. Have your bike checked

Biking might be related to low sperm count. Bicycling more than five hours per week is associated with lower sperm concentration. Having your bike checked for a proper fit can help.

7. Wear loose, cotton boxers

Keeping your sperm at an adequate temperature and allowing lots of air flow to the scrotum can help cultivate the right environment for healthy sperm. If you don't feel comfortable wearing boxers, choose cotton briefs instead of synthetic ones. That will still help control air flow and temperature.

Healthy sperm

Sperm count isn't the only thing that matters when trying to conceive. You also want to have overall healthy sperm.

A male's reproductive health is defined by three aspects of sperm:

1. the health of the individual sperm

2. the amount or concentration of sperm

3. the volume of the overall sperm

Some findings suggest that men's sperm quality is declining. Doctors aren't completely sure why that is happening, but lifestyle and nutrition may play a role.

Does sperm count affect IVF success?

Sperm count affects the use of reproductive technology, such as in vitro fertilization (IVF), as well. Your success in using IVF with a low sperm count will depend on the health of your sperm and what factors are causing the low sperm count. The sperm can now be injected directly into the egg through a process called intracytoplasmic sperm injection as an alternative if the man has a very low sperm count.

No matter how you are hoping to conceive, improving your sperm count can help improve your chances of a successful pregnancy.

When to see a doctor

The common advice given to couples trying to conceive is to see a doctor after one year of unprotected sex that does not result in pregnancy. If the female partner is over 35, see a doctor after six months of unprotected sex that does not result in a pregnancy.

If you have a known occupation, hobby, or medical condition that is linked to a lower sperm count, you should talk to a doctor as soon as possible before you begin trying to conceive. They can do tests to ensure that you're healthy and conception is recommended.

If you're having trouble conceiving, a fertility specialist will usually perform tests on both the man and woman. A woman will have her eggs, ovaries, and uterus tested. A man will provide a semen sample for a semen analysis and sperm count. The doctor will check the number of sperm per sample to determine if the sperm count is too low. An ultrasound may also be performed to look for problems in the scrotum, or ducts and tubes where the semen travels.

Outlook

The success rate of achieving pregnancy with a low sperm count will vary based on your and your partner's individual health. If you decide you want to have a family, there are many options available to you, such as pursuing adoption, exploring IVF, or making lifestyle changes to try to conceive. Your first step is talking with a doctor who can help assess sperm count and other fertility factors before making a plan for your future.

Can Nux Vomica Treat Male Infertility?

What is nux vomica?

Nux vomica is commonly used as a natural remedy for many different symptoms and disorders. It comes from an evergreen tree by the same name, which is native to China, East India, Thailand, and Australia. The raw seeds are nicknamed "poison nut" because of their toxic nature. They must be treated before they are consumed to make them safe. Nux vomica that is used as a supplement can be purchased in a pill or powder form.

Nux vomica can affect the nervous system, and is most often used to treat conditions that are acute, or develop rapidly and have a short course. It is sometimes used to treat erectile dysfunction and infertility in men, though actual scientific studies have not yet proven its effectiveness.

Benefits of nux vomica

Some people believe that nux vomica has anti-inflammatory properties. Anti-inflammatories are used to treat conditions that are worsened by inflammation, such as rheumatism, asthma, or hemorrhoids. One study found that nux vomica was effective in reducing the inflammation in rat paws.

Studies have shown that nux vomica contains powerful antioxidants. Antioxidants protect you against free radicals, which are chemicals in your body that can damage your cells.

The flowers of nux vomica are also believed to have antibacterial properties. According to one study, these properties could potentially be beneficial for use in antiseptics. Further research needs to be conducted.

What does nux vomica treat?

Nux vomica is used to treat many different conditions. These include:

- digestive problems such as constipation, bloating, heartburn, and nausea

- male infertility and impotence

- colds and flus, particularly in the early stages of the virus

- allergies

- back pain

- irritability, impatience, and high sensitivity to stimuli, caused by stress or mental strain

- headaches and migraines symptoms such as a sore scalp, frontal pain, light sensitivity, or stomach problems

- hangovers

- menstrual problems

- insomnia

At this time, there isn't much scientific evidence that nux vomica effectively treats these symptoms and conditions. Talk to your doctor before you start using nux vomica. They may recommend other medications to treat your condition or symptoms, or may know of other, more effective homeopathic remedies to try first.

Who should avoid nux vomica?

You shouldn't use nux vomica if you have liver disease, as it can cause liver damage.

Nux vomica shouldn't be taken in high doses, or used as a long-term treatment. Taking too much can cause serious symptoms, including:

- restlessness

- anxiety

- dizziness

- back stiffness

- liver failure

- breathing problems

- seizures

The potential neurologic side effects of nux vomica are very serious. Because of this, the Centers for Disease Control and Prevention list nux vomica as a chemical hazard.

You should consult your doctor before using nux vomica to treat male infertility or erectile dysfunction. They can help determine the underlying cause of the issue, and offer more effective treatments.

Tell your doctor about all of the medications you're taking. Nux vomica can cause dangerous drug interactions, especially with antipsychotics.

It's also important to note that while nux vomica has antioxidants, which are beneficial to overall health, taking antioxidants in doses that are too high can result in health problems.

Takeaway

Nux vomica has been used throughout history as a natural supplement to treat impotency and male infertility, along with many other conditions. However, there is no substantial evidence that it is effective.

The potentially toxic properties of nux vomica and its side effects are not worth the risk when other treatments

are available.